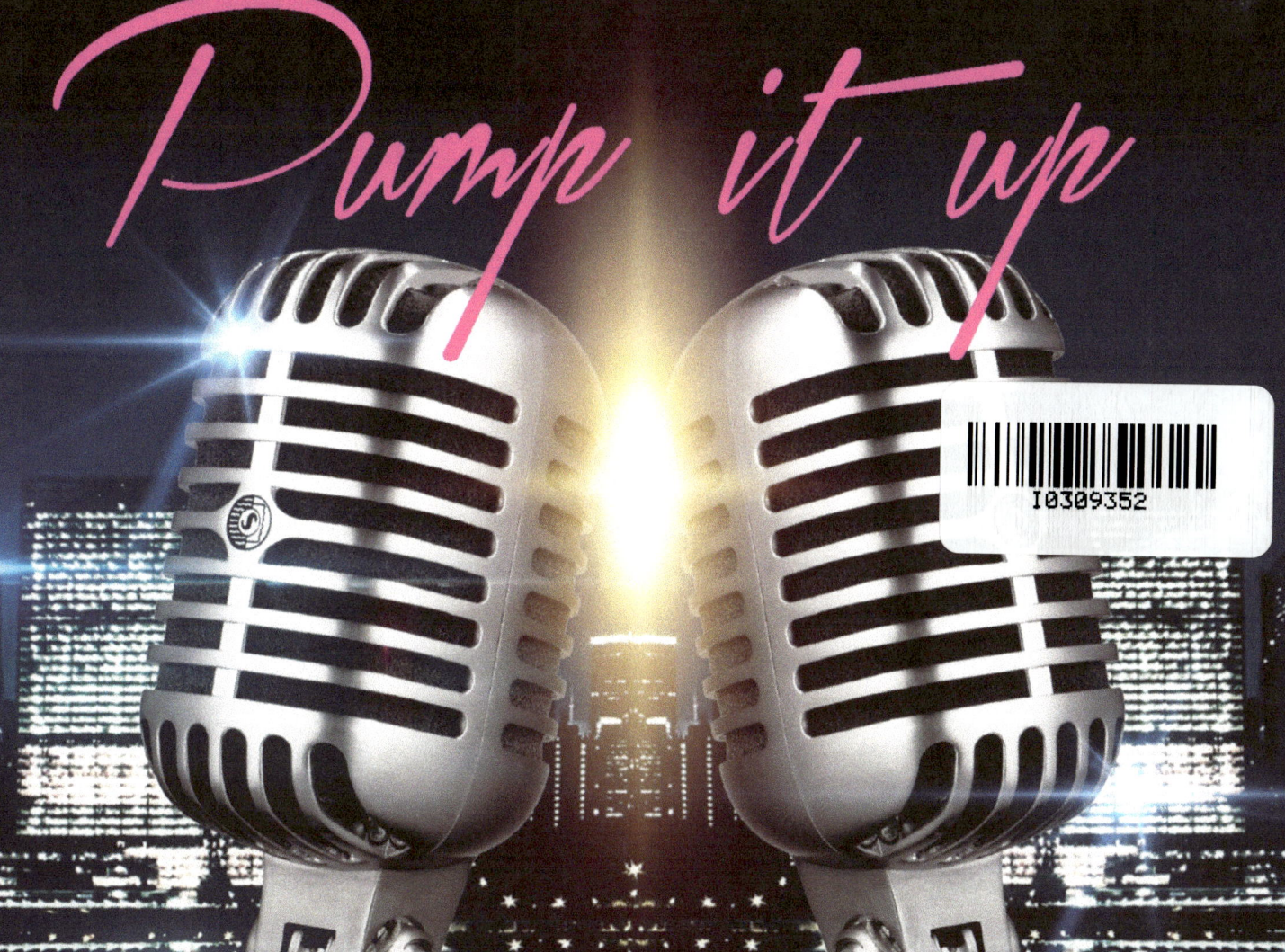

Pump it up Magazine

TABLE OF CONTENTS

DAMIAN HASBUN
Bringing Life Out of The Music!

EDITORIAL 6
Page 5

HAPPY INDEPENDENCE DAY
- Celebrating America With Our Favorite Patriotic Songs
- Summer NAAM 2021
- Books To Read This Summer

REVIEW 11
The Future of Music Technology

BEAUTY
What is Microneedling facial?

STYLE 21
Shades, Shoes, And Dresses

TOP TIPS
How To Become A Better Singer

MUST WATCH 28
"Old" By M. Shyamalan

HUMANITARIAN AWARENESS
Help Raise PTSD Awareness

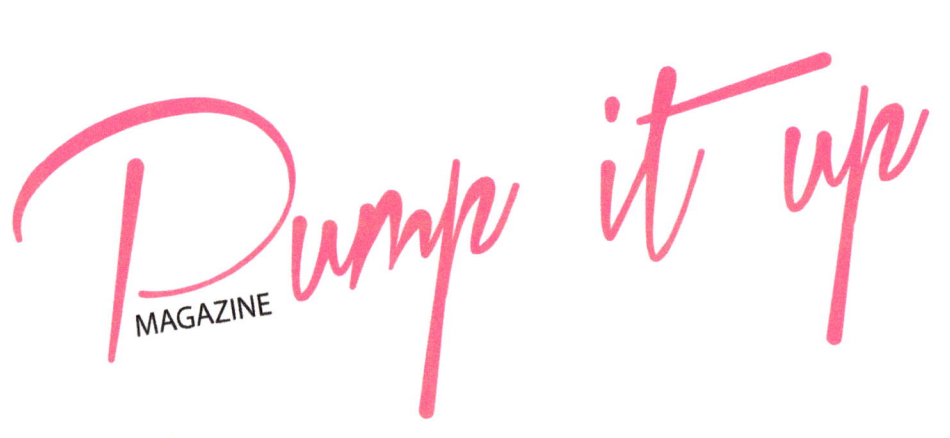
Pump it up
MAGAZINE

PUMP IT UP MAGAZINE
LINKS

WEBSITE
www.pumpitupmagazine.com

FACEBOOK
www.facebook.com/pumpitupmagazine

TWITTER
www.twitter.com/pumpitupmag

SOUNDCLOUD
www.soundcloud.com/pumpitupmagazine

INSTAGRAM
pumpitupmagazine

PINTEREST
www.pinterest.com/pumpitupmagazine

PUMP IT UP MAGAZINE
30721 Russell Ranch Road
Suite 140
Westlake Village,
California 91362
United States
www.pumpitupmagazine.com
info@pumpitupmagazine.com
Tel : (001) (877)841 – 7414 (toll free number)

EDITORIAL

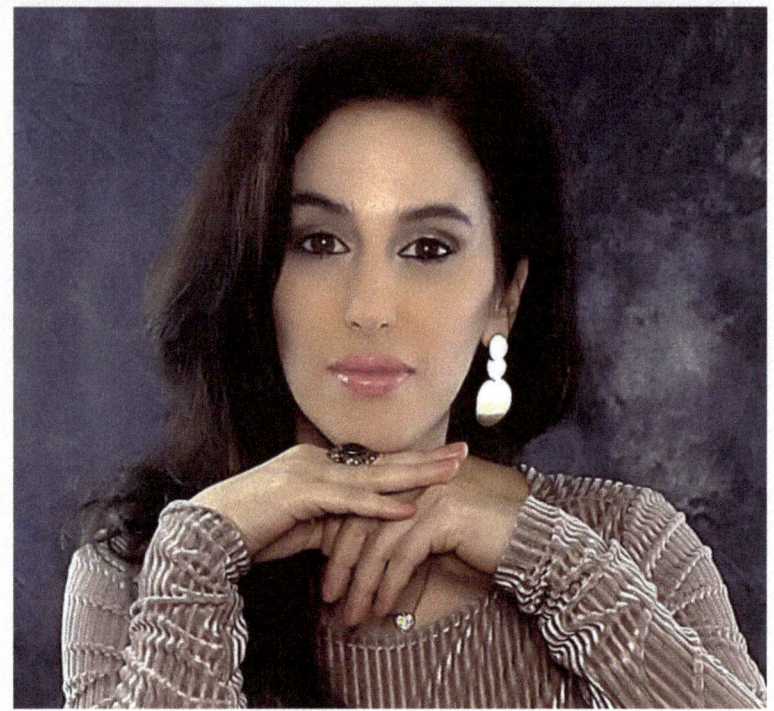

Greetings,

Happy Fourth of July Readers.

Summer is officially here so fire up the barby this weekend and pick up the latest issue of Pump It Up Magazine, sit back and flip thru the pages while the coals are heating.

On the cover we have renowned sound engineer Damian Hasbun of Evenform Studio.

Damian Hasbun is an engineer who has worked with the likes of DMX and French Montana.

In the issues we also explore the introduction of AI (artificial intelligence) in music.

Don't forget to check out page 16 and see our collection of 4th of. July jams!

Not to mention our usual coverage of the latest in fashion, literature and film.

Our pages are full of information that will inspire, promote positivity, and more.

Each edition we feature our Humanitarian Awareness page. This issue we want to raise PTSD awareness.

Please don't forget to tune in to Pump It Up Magazine Radio where you will hear the best of indie and major artists.'

Be well, be safe!

Anissa Boudjaoui

CONTRIBUTORS

EDITOR IN CHIEF
Anissa Boudjaoui

MUSIC
Michael B. Sutton
A. Scott Galloway
Sarah Kaye

FASHION
Tiffani Sutton

MARKETING
Grace Rose

PARTNERS

Editions L.A.
www.editions-la.com

The Sound Of L.A.
www.thesoundofla.com

Info Music
www.infomusic.fr

Delit Face
www.DelitFace.com

L.A. Unlimited
www.launlimitedinc.com

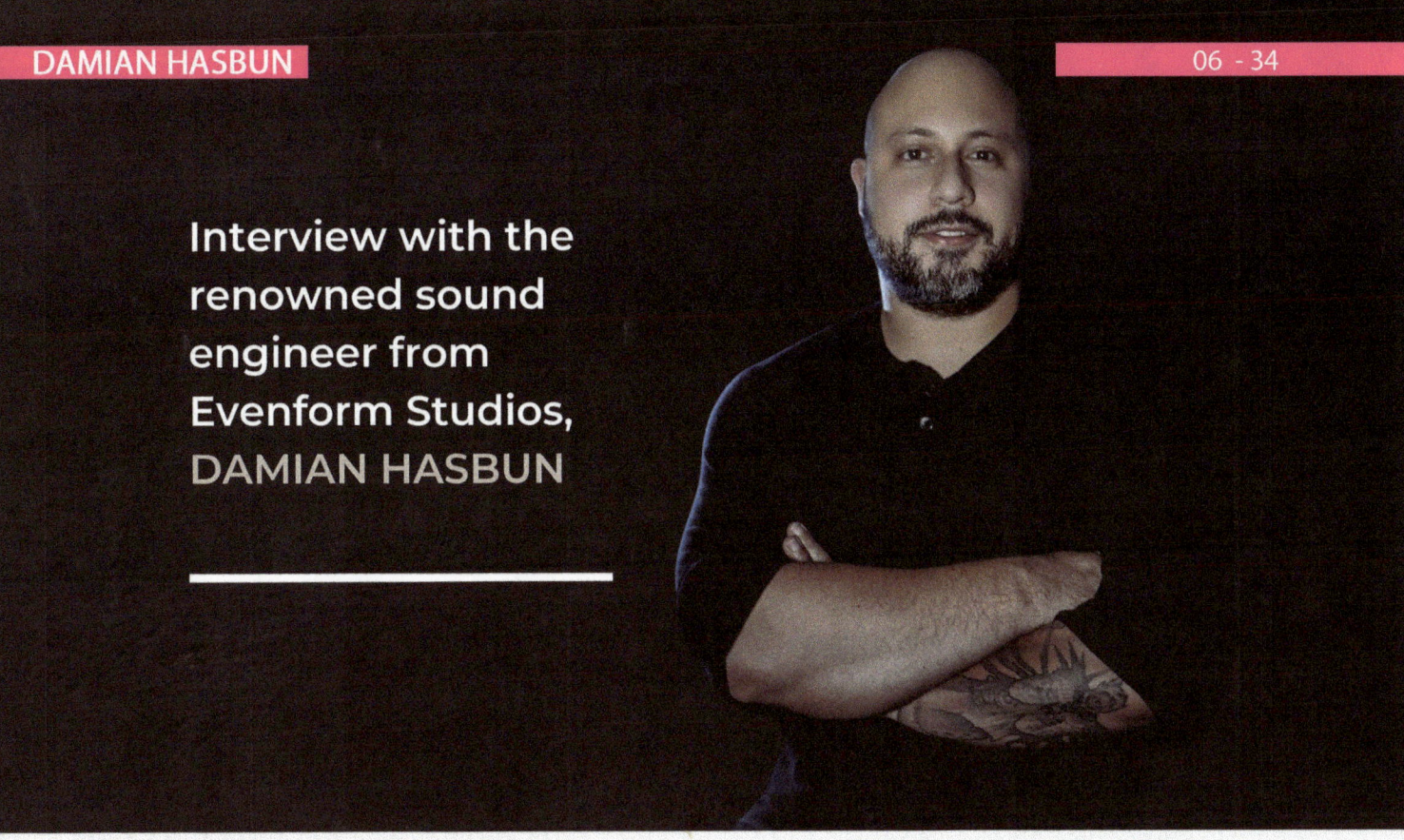

Interview with the renowned sound engineer from Evenform Studios, DAMIAN HASBUN

We held an interview with the renowned sound engineer from Evenform Studios, Damian Hasbun. Damian is an apprentice of the owner and founder of Evenform Studios, Jesse Clark whom he has been a fan of long before knowing him. Damian is now under the mentorship of King James, who has worked with names like Diddy, Debaby, Notorious BIG, Keyshia Cole, Complex TV and BET.

Damian knew from his high school days that his career would be something involving music as he had a strong desire to surround himself with the art of music. Damian's first gig was with Evenform Studios in Raleigh NC. Since then, he has worked with a collective of various artists. Damian's biggest achievement according to him, was to engineer A Flock of Seagulls latest album, Ascension. As Evenform works with names like DMX and French Montana, Mr. Hasbun is fortunate enough to be in the position to work with a great clientele. Damian mostly finds his work through client recommendations. Working for the largest recording studio in the city with a 5 star rating and 15 year long history do help too. His favorite DAW is Protools though he grew up using FL Studio. In his words,

"I see myself as a musical scientist, and I play the role of a psychological motivator. Taking on projects to mix and master are always a joy to me. I'm truly passionate about my work and I love a great challenge!"

According to Damian, great sound engineers are able to make the listener feel the soul of the music. Some songs require a more skilled sound engineer to make them sound the way they're intended to sound on a spiritual level. He loves working on songs that are emotional and have an element of dance to it. Even if it's a sad dance. In Damian's opinion, a good mix and master means that the mission is complete and no further changes need to be made. The listener should feel the magic the artist has created.

Currently, Mr. Hasbun is working with an artist named Shame Gang. They've completed an album called No Safe Haven.

For Mixing and Mastering quotes email your sessions to Damianhasbun@yahoo.com
Please visit: http://evenformstudio.com/

DAMIAN HASBUN

1. TELL US A LITTLE BIT ABOUT THE DAY-TO-DAY LIFE OF A SOUND ENGINEER

I see myself as a musical scientist, and I play the role of a psychological motivator. Taking on projects to mix and master are always a joy to me. I'm truly passionate about my work and I love a great challenge!

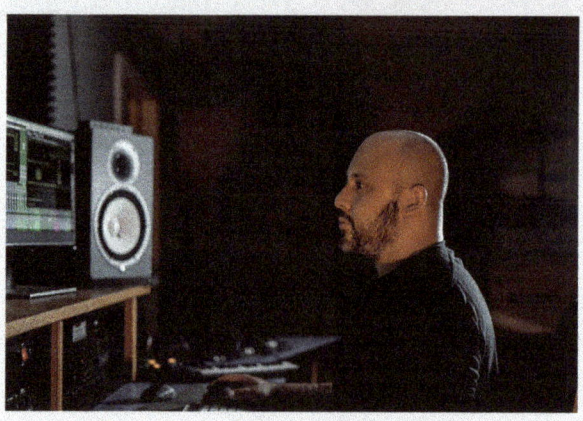

2. WHO ARE SOME OF THE ARTISTS YOU'VE WORKED WITH?

I've worked with a lot of great artists over the years but I would have to say my biggest achievement was working with the band A Flock Of Seagulls. I was lucky enough to be one of the engineers of their latest album "Ascension".
This was the first time my parents said they were proud when it came to my career as an engineer haha.
They were huge fans growing up. The studio I work for, Evenform, has worked with the biggest artists in the world from DMX, French Montana to Alesana, so i've been incredibly fortunate to have found myself in the position to work the great clientele they provide me.

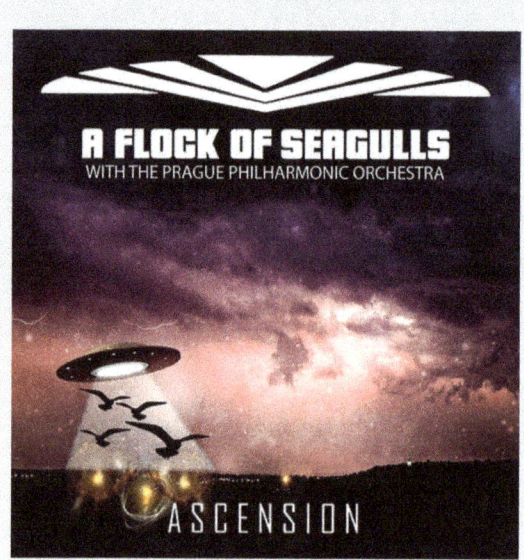

3. WHAT KIND OF TRAINING DO YOU HAVE?

Initially my training had begun from learning under Jesse Clark, Evenform owner and founder. Before knowing who he was, I used to listen to his productions and were amazed by the musicality of the records he had worked on. My mentor now Is King James who has worked with countless big artists such as Biggie Smalls and P Diddy. It's been such an honor to be able to learn under people I look up to and respect.

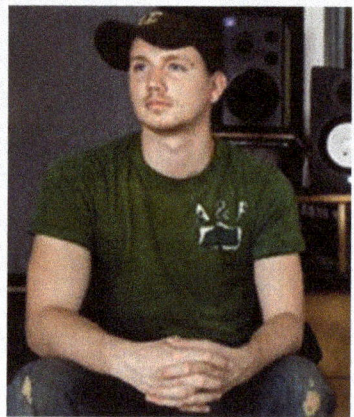

Jesse Clark

4. WHEN DID YOU KNOW YOU WANTED TO BECOME A SOUND ENGINEER?

I didn't know I was going to be a sound engineer but I always knew that my career would be involved in creating music. Since high school I had such a strong desire to surround myself with the art of music and I've always been extremely competitive. It is definitely my calling.

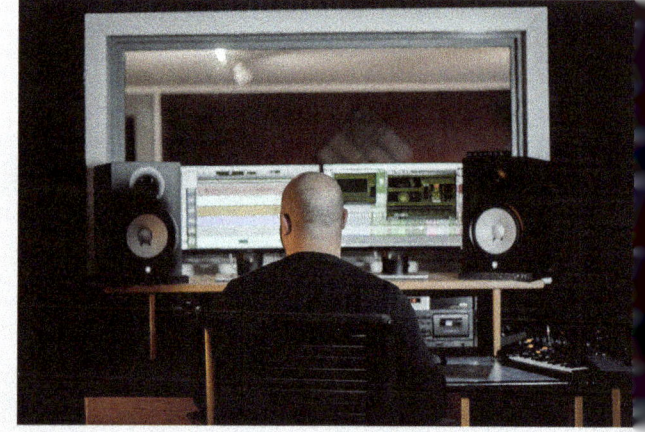

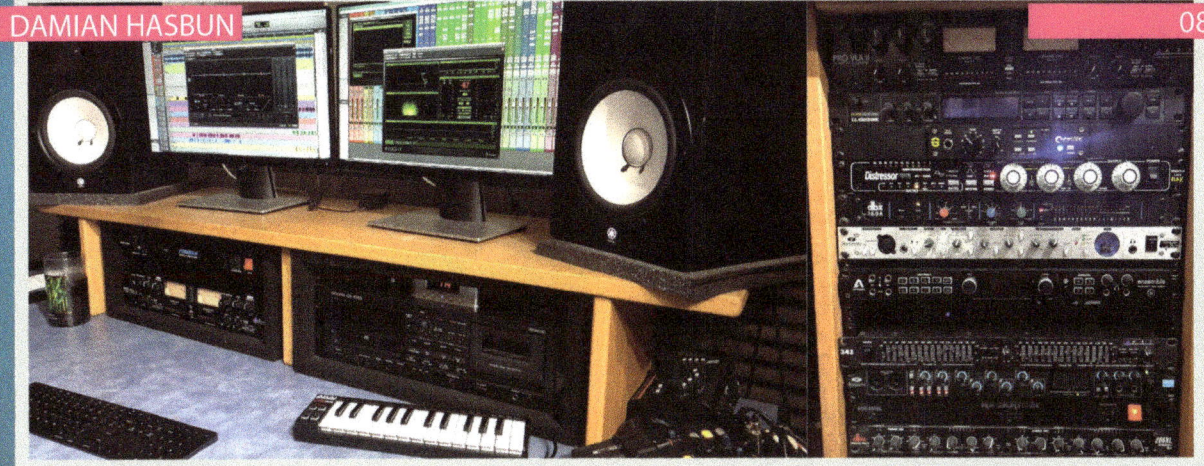

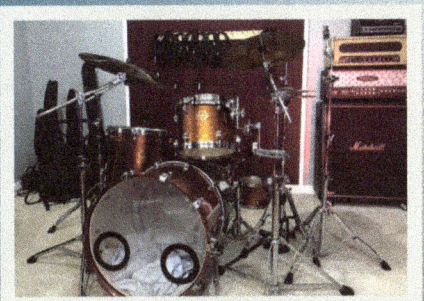

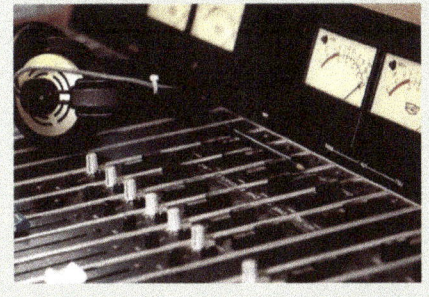

EVENFORM RECORDING STUDIO

EVENFORM RECORDING STUDIO
809 N. WEST STREET
RALEIGH, NC 27603
(919) 398-1825
EVENFORMSTUDIO.COM

5. HOW DID YOU GET YOUR FIRST SR GIG

Evenform Studios in Raleigh NC gave me my first gig. Ever since then it's been uphill for me and I'm extremely grateful!

6. HOW DO YOU FIND WORK?

I find most of my work through word of mouth and client recommendation. It also helps that the studio I work for is the highest rated recording studio in my city. We are rated 5 Star and have been around for over 15 years so we have a long history.

7. WHAT SEPARATES A GOOD SOUND ENGINEER FROM A BAD ONE?

I don't believe in good sound engineers. I believe in great sound engineers. Great sound engineers are able to make the listener feel the soul of the music. Some songs require a more skilled sound engineer to bring the life out of the music. That's where my role comes into play. I'm the person they hire to bring the music to life and make it sound the way it's intended to sound on a spiritual level.

8. WHAT WOULD BE THE MAJOR REASONS TO GO INTO YOUR PROFESSIONAL STUDIO (EVENFORM) OVER A HOME-RECORDING SET-UP?

Hmm, I mean technically if an artist wanted me to record in a bathroom I would. Maybe even in a haunted house, I would find that cool and interesting. I wouldn't be able to bring all the expensive gear that Evenform has at the studio though haha

9. ANY SPECIFIC GENRE OF MUSIC YOU LIKE TO WORK ON – DO YOU ACCEPT ANY GENRES?

I'm not picky with genre but I love working on songs that are emotional and have an element of dance to it. Even if it's a sad dance where you just nod your head. Absolutely love those!

YOUR MUSIC CONSULTANT

"YOU BELIEVE, SO DO WE!"

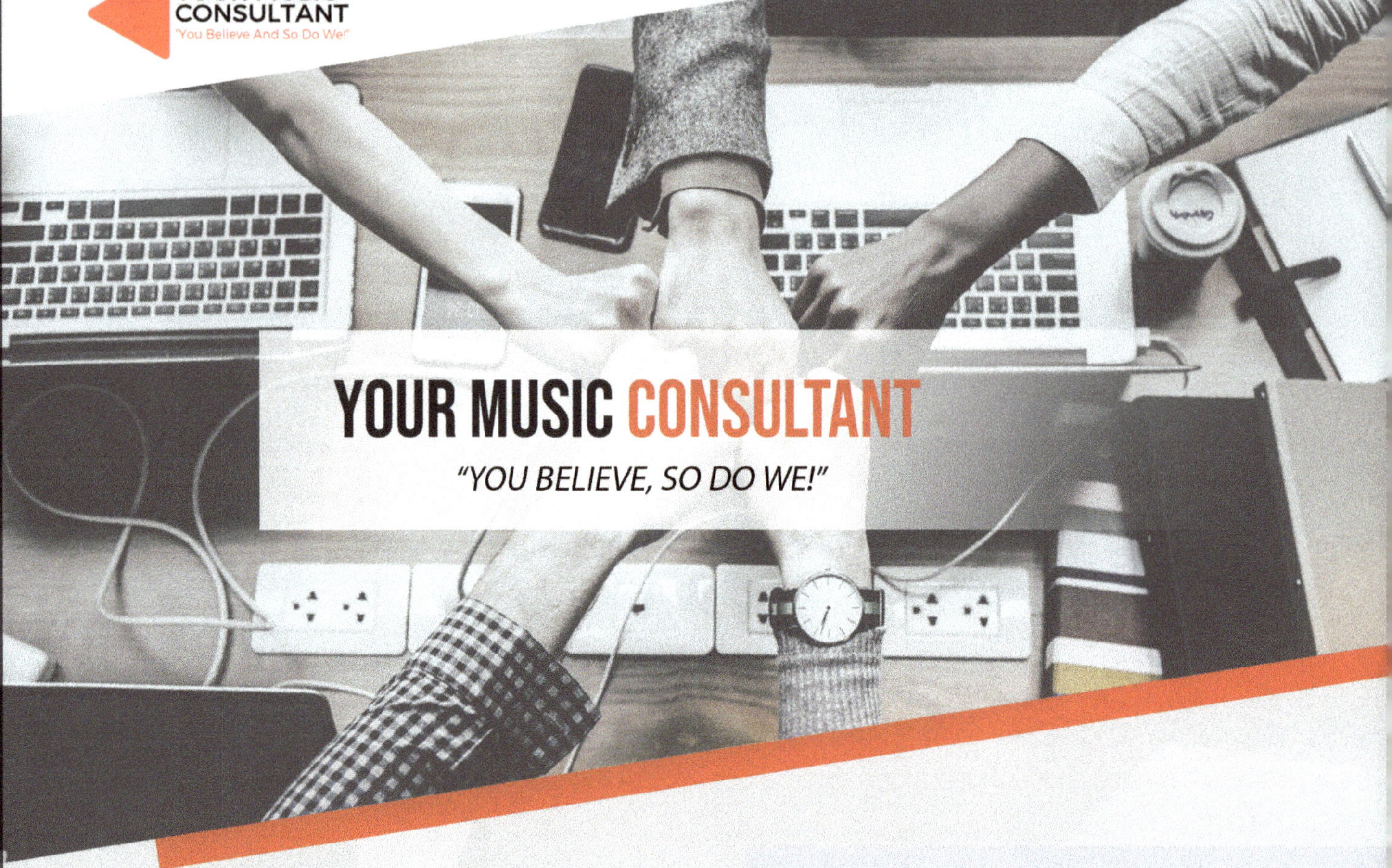

We Can Help You To Grow Your Business

We are a monthly based service, we put faith in artists who has major potential, believed in them, and who are willing to spend their time and own money to work with us in building a successful music career!

Digital Marketing Services
SOCIAL MEDIA - STREAMING SERVICES - MUSIC DISTRIBUTION - PRESS RELEASE - PRESS DISTRIBUTION - PR

Radio Airplay and TV Commercial
TERRESTRIAL AND DIGITAL RADIO CAMPAIGN AL GENRES EXCEPT HEAVY METAL - CABLE TV AND MAJOR NETWORK COMMERCIAL

Licensing & Booking
CONCERTS, LIVE MUSIC, EVENTS, CLUB NIGHTS - RED CARPETS - FOREIGN LICENSING AND SUBOPUBLISHING

Why Choose Us ?

3 DECADES OF MUSIC BUSINESS EXPERIENCE
Platinum and Gold Records
MOTOWN RECORDS
UNIVERSAL
SONY
CAPITOL RECORDS

WE WORKED WITH:
Kanye West - Jay Z - Stevie Wonder - Michael Jackson - Germaine Jackson - Smokey Robinson - Dionne Warwick - Cheryl Lynn - The Originals -

📞 1 -818-514-0038
(Ext. 1)
Monday - Friday / 9am to 6pm

FIND US :

www.YourMusicConsultant.com
30721 Russell Ranch Road Suite 140 Westlake Village, USA
Email : info@yourmusicconsultant.com

EDITIONS L.A.

GRAPHIC AND WEB **DESIGN**

WEBSITE
CD COVER
LOGO
FLYER
BANNERS
EPK
LYRICS VIDEO
TRANSLATION

We give you the tools to make your song or band to be heard around the world!

INFO@ EDITIONS-L.A.COM

WWW.EDITIONS-LA.COM

SPECIAL **OFFERS** 50% ON LYRICS VIDEOS
HIGH-QUALITY MUSIC LYRICS VIDEO
UP TO 1080P HD VIDEO QUALITY
MODERN AND SIMPLE STYLE
$250 FOR MUSIC VIDEO UP TO 4 MIN
$350 FOR MUSIC VIDEO UP TO 5 MIN

FOR MORE INFO VISIT WWW.EDITIONS-LA.COM

THE FUTURE OF MUSIC WITH AI

AI. Artificial intelligence. Those unfamiliar have at least seen it demonstrated in Hollywood – I, Robot, Terminator 3: Rise of the Machines, Bicentennial Man, Spielberg's aptly named, A.I. Artificial Intelligence, the list goes on.
One area seeing an increasingly larger presence of AI is in the music industry, with its effects felt across the creation, promotion, application, and listening processes.

AI and machine learning are changing the very face of the music industry, from the way music is made to its consumption, but is it all for the better?

AI IN THE MUSIC INDUSTRY: MAJOR OR MINOR IMPROVEMENT?
The music industry at large is not immune to the growing presence of AI in the general workforce.

True to the "augment vs. replace" distinction, it is expected that music producer and songwriter jobs will be augmented, rather than outright replaced, as AI continues to integrate into the creative process.

AI technologies and applications have become significantly more popular and capable, increasing data volumes and advancing algorithms while providing improvements in computing power and storage, all commodities that music creators need.

While innovations in how we create music and how it is consumed are indeed exciting, as a creator, one must be wary of completely removing the human element out of art. Because, naturally, all art forms are, by definition, human.

Music is littered with notions of subjectivity and taste; it's a transaction with emotional currency, so it is difficult to wrap my head around a computer being able to tap into the creative process, as well as the intellectual components that make great music resonate.

In Bicentennial Man, they had to make Robin Williams fully human before he could really be human. I think this says a lot about AI's role in music and the arts in general.

Below, I outline several innovations in the world of AI in music, and speak to a few pros and cons that I've observed.

AI = THE NEW MUSICIAN?
Over the last several decades, there are numerous examples of musicians using AI-generated methods like neural networks to fuel the creative process and augment music composition. These have run the gamut from more boutique, "techy" offerings, to Billboard-charting singles.

In 2016, super producer Alex da Kid released the song "Not Easy," a collaboration with X-Ambassadors, Elle King, Wiz Khalifa and…IBM's computer system, "Watson." Said Rolling Stone, "Watson…presented five years of analyzed cultural data in a way that meant something to Alex: through colors, patterns, textures, and words, Alex was able to read the data in a customized way – a data visualization made up of colors, words, patterns, and textures – that moved him."

In 2017, American Idol alum Taryn Southern released I AM AI, an album that's music was composed entirely by an AI composition program from Amper Music that used internal algorithms to produce melodies that blended appropriately with a particular mood and genre.

EXAMPLES OF AI IN MUSIC

AI CASE STUDY #1: SHAZAM

Perhaps one of the most stunning innovations in the world of artificial intelligence is one that sits neatly on our phones: Shazam.

One of the first consumer-adopted artificial intelligence services, Shazam uses intelligent technology to listen to and then identify songs, all in a matter of seconds. How many times have you been to a bar or restaurant and seen someone randomly holding up their arm with their phone in their hand, or even standing on a chair to get it closer to a speaker?

Partnering with Apple Music, Shazam does the equivalent of a fingerprint or retina scan on a piece of music. It matches that scan to the Apple Music library and swiftly comes up with the song. The song is then automatically added to the user's Apple Music library under the pre-made "My Shazam Tracks" playlist.

I can't tell you the number of times I have been watching television shows like The O.C., Shameless, Bojack Horseman or Insecure and thought, "Wow! That's a great song! I wonder what that is?!" then held my phone to the TV and voila! there it is, loaded onto my phone ready for listening.

Shazam's service provides an incredible amount of consumer satisfaction, and it very well may be my favorite piece of artificial intelligence technology that exists.

AI CASE STUDY #2: MUSIC STREAMING SERVICES & PLAYLISTING

Streaming services are now the dominant force in all aspects of music, overtaking digital downloads as the next big thing.

Spotify's bread-and-butter is their "Discover Weekly" playlists. These are generated for users based on an algorithm that reacts to a user's listening history and creates a playlist highlighting their tastes, as well as new music that the algorithm thinks they will like.

Spotify's artificial intelligence undergoes ongoing improvements by collecting as much listening data as possible, performing a comparative analysis from other users, and then uses these results to suggest new music.

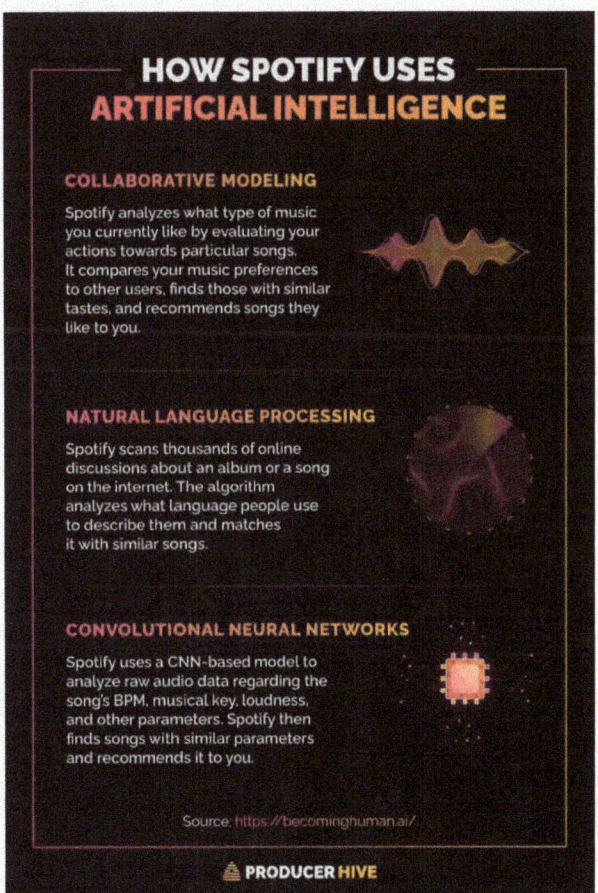

Apple Music is different because, as it claims, their playlists are strictly curated by an expert curation team. Additionally, one of Apple's flagship services is Apple Music 1 Radio – formerly Beats 1 Radio – which is a 24-hour radio service that is curated and hosted by actual DJs and celebrity hosts.

Despite the convenience of Spotify's machine learning/algorithm-centric playlists, Apple Music's human curation provides a personal touch to the music discovery process. Additionally, Apple Music will inform playlist subscribers when a playlist has been updated with new music.

AI CASE STUDY #3: LANDR

The final area I would like to particularly focus on is artificial intelligence in music production. AI audio mastering services are beginning to seize major market share from traditional mastering engineers, with the major player being LANDR. But to better understand this competition, we need to answer a simple question: what exactly is mastering?

Mastering makes your completed music sound professional, balanced, cohesive, and competitive for commercial release, while ensuring that it maintains the same level of quality across a wide variety of speaker systems and media formats.

This is done through the following processes, via Icon Collective:

Emphasizing or reducing certain frequencies
Fix phase – out-of-sync soundwave – issues
Create an even distribution of frequencies to help dynamic recordings translate on different playback systems, protecting against low-end rumble and harsh high-end
Remove pops, clicks, and other unwanted noises from a sound source
So how does LANDR work? Straight from the horse's mouth, LANDR uses machine learning to replicate the "human intelligence" mastering process through "smart" mastering software that is…

"Built around an adaptive engine that 'listens' and reacts to music, using micro-genre detection to make subtle frame-by-frame adjustments using tools like multi-band compression, EQ, stereo enhancement, limiting and harmonic saturation, based on the unique properties of your song."

Having the ability to finish a song, then have it mastered in a matter of minutes, all without having to leave your chair or deal with communication channels, various schedules, and invoicing, is pretty amazing.

But here's the thing. No matter how smart LANDR's software may be, it makes decisions based on algorithms, not emotions or feelings.

Inevitably, this can result in just-OK-sounding masters, however, if you are only paying $20/song, can you really be that upset?

Mastering engineers, however, can respond on instinct and feeling, can go through several rounds of feedback, while also having the ability to master a full album, complete with consistent loudness levels from track-to-track, fades, etc.

AI just can't match that level of personal intimacy… for now.

AI IS HERE TO STAY, BUT ITS CONTRIBUTIONS ARE A GREY AREA

So as has been outlined, artificial intelligence is an ever-populating tool that can be utilized in most industries. Its contributions to music composition, production and more, are farther-reaching by the year.

But how long before legalities come into play?

With current copyright law as it stands, currently, there is nothing to legally stand in the way of AI copying an artists' style, inflections, and instincts. Some legal experts say that unless the AI is directly sampling, being directly marketed as sounding like that particular artist, or creating derivative works, then there is nothing to be done.

SUMMER NAAM 2021

>>>>>>>>>>>

Summer NAMM will return to Nashville and the Music City Center, July 15–16, 2021.

A Summer NAMM badge includes:
Access to hundreds of brands
Free professional education at NAMM U and TEC Tracks
Complimentary entrance to Top 100 Dealer Awards
Exclusive rates at official Summer NAMM hotels
Discounts on flights and ground transportation
Deals at restaurants & attractions around Nashville
Assistance for international travelers requiring a visa
Access to thousands of influencers, ideas and new opportunities

WWW.NAMM.ORG <<<<<<<<<<<

DELIT FACE

Social Media For The Entertainment World

MUSIC & MOVIE Industry

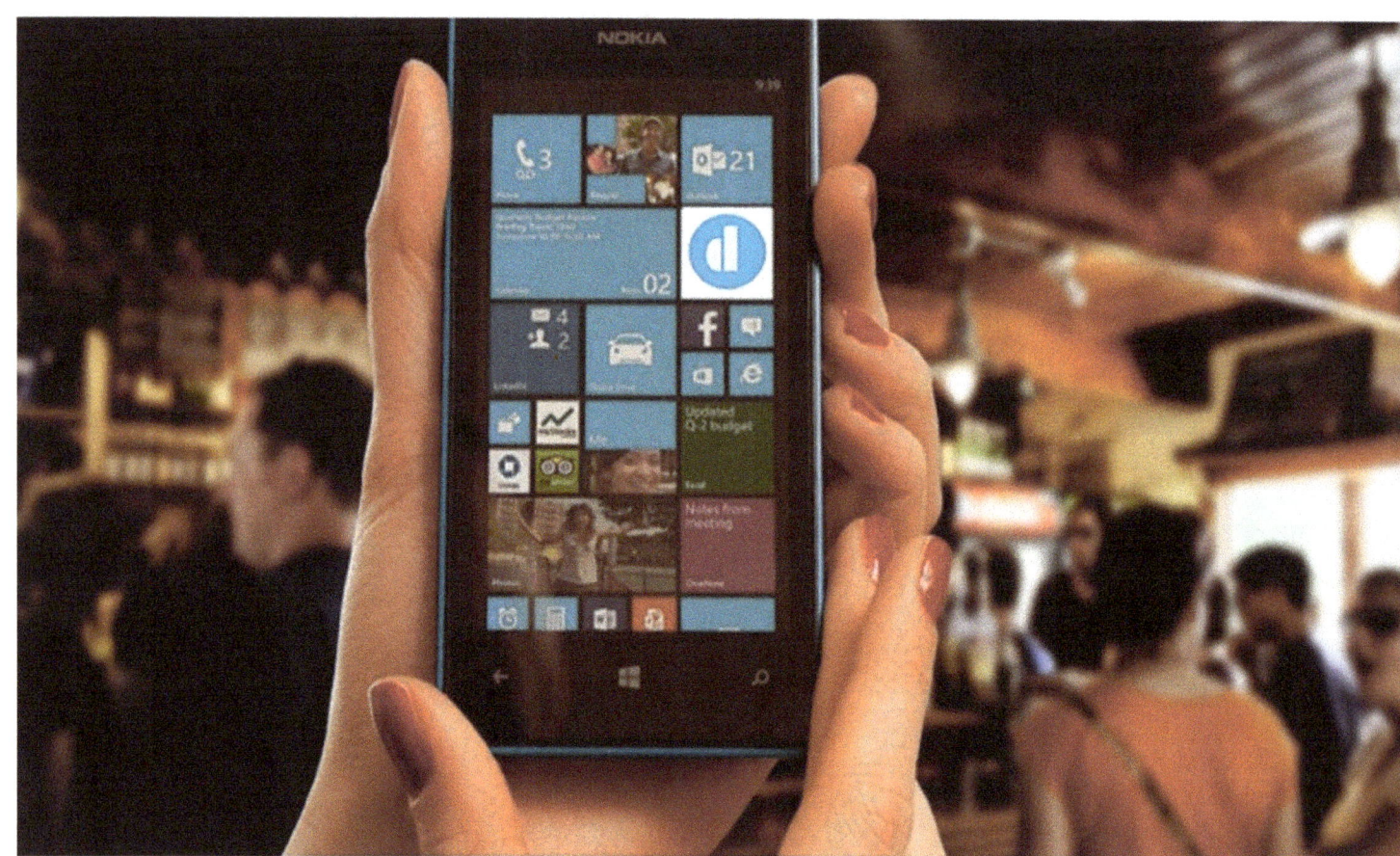

SINGER
SONGWRITER
MUSICIANS
PRODUCERS
PUBLISHERS
DISTRIBUTORS
MUSIC SUPERVISORS

ACTORS
DIRECTORS
PRODUCERS
DISTRIBUTORS
SET DESIGNERS
SCRIPT WRITERS
EXTRAS

MAKE UP ARTISTS
HAIR STYLISTS
PHOTOGRAPHERS
GRAPHIC DESIGNER

Register now FREE and connect with people in your industry
www.delitface.com

PUMP IT UP MAGAZINE
MUSIC SELECTION

★ ★ ★

FOURTH OF JULY
Celebration

SUN **04** JULY

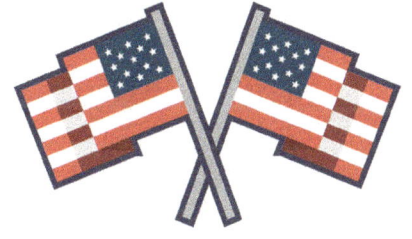

OUR FAVORITE PATRIOTIC SONGS

@pumpitupmagazine

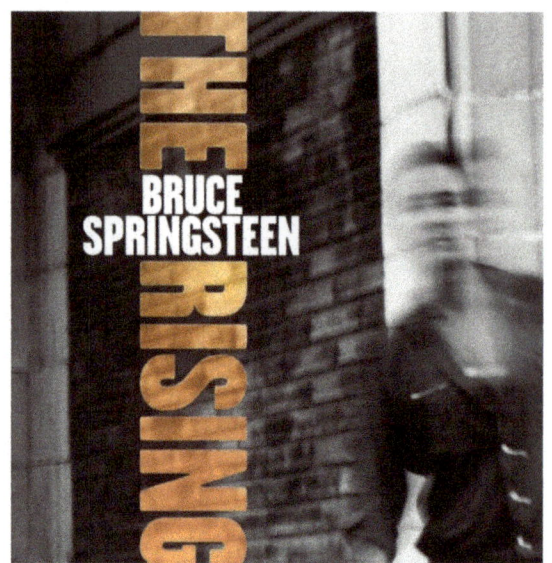

Bruce Springsteen: My City of Ruins

Originally written about Asbury Park, New Jersey, when Bruce Springsteen performed the song as part of the America: A Tribute to Heroes benefit concert, it instantly became a patriotic anthem deeply connected to New York and September 11th. – Sam Armstrong

X: 4th Of July

"4th Of July" was the only song Blasters guitarist Dave Alvin contributed to the LA punk pioneers' 1987 album, See How We Are. As one of the more unconventional 4th of July songs, it's a gritty triumph about a love affair on the skids that makes a last-ditch attempt to get back on track so the couple can celebrate a little. A blue-collar anthem if there ever was one. – Brett Milano

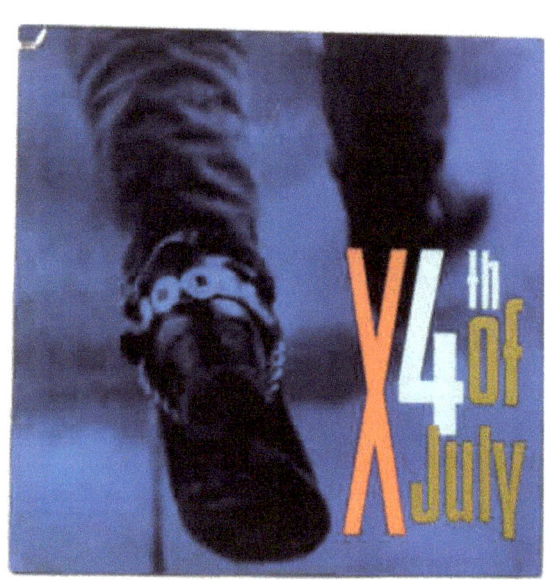

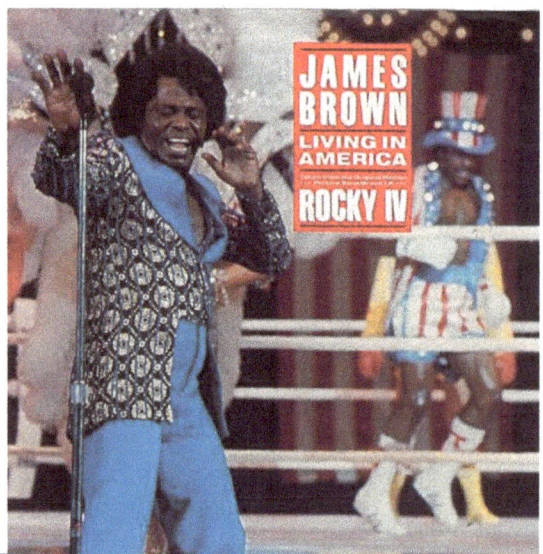

James Brown: Living In America

Perhaps inevitably, it was James Brown (and songwriter Dan Hartman) who came up with a song that everybody in America, no matter their political beliefs or lifestyle, could get down to. Sometimes you've just gotta have a celebration to the funkiest of all patriotic songs. – Brett Milano

BOOKS | 18 - 34

Best Beach Reads

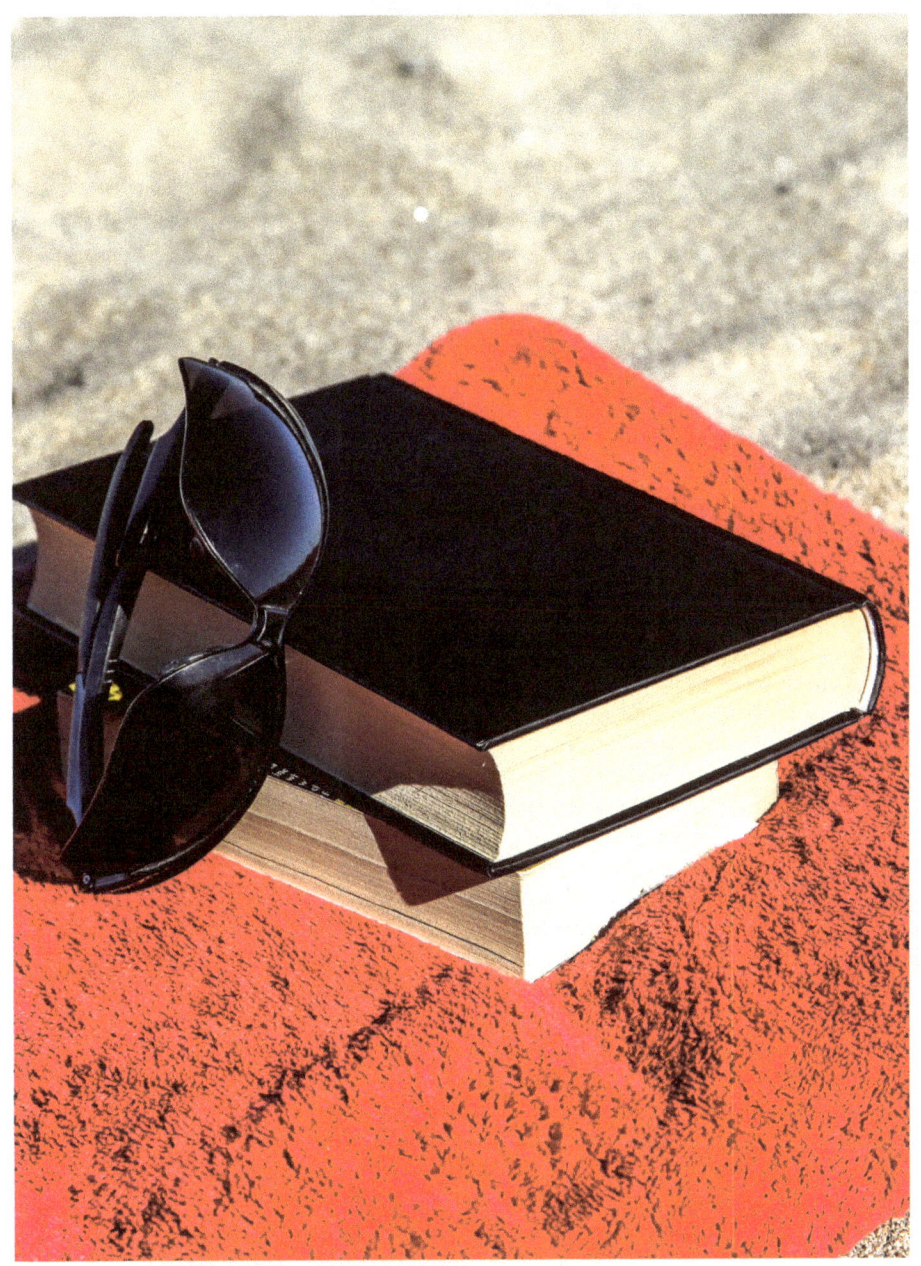

BOOKS TO READ THIS SUMMER

BOOKS

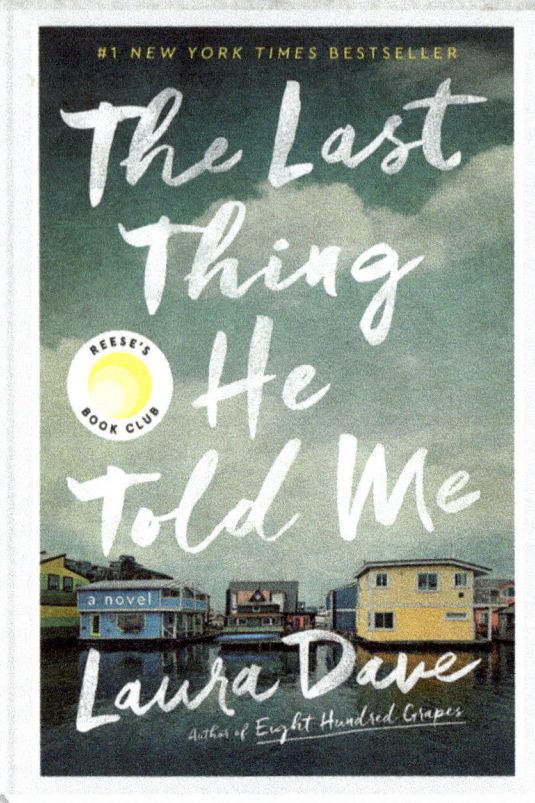
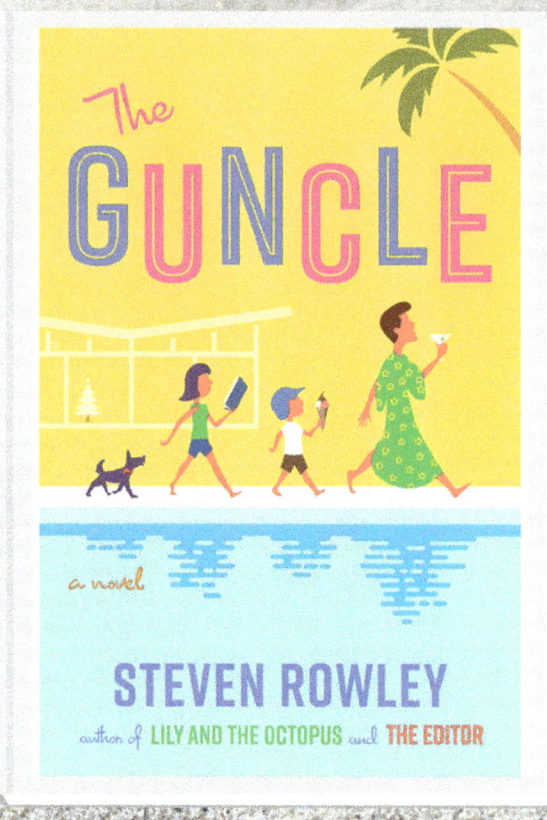
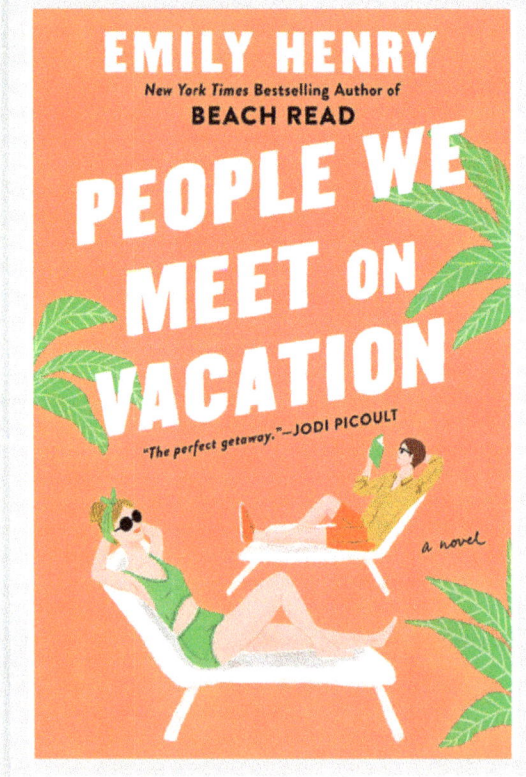
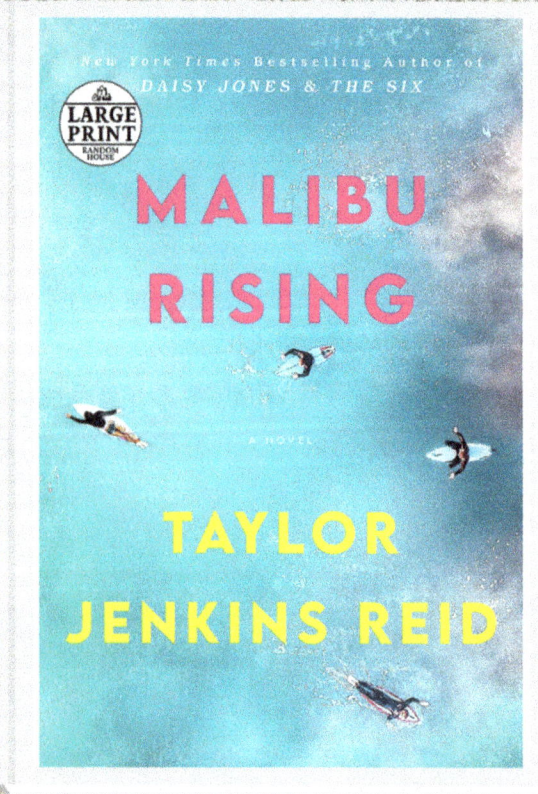

Are you a songwriter or composer struggling to protect your work and releases?
Well Bernie Capodici has done all the work for you in his new book
"Modern Recording Artist Handbook, How To Guide Simplified"

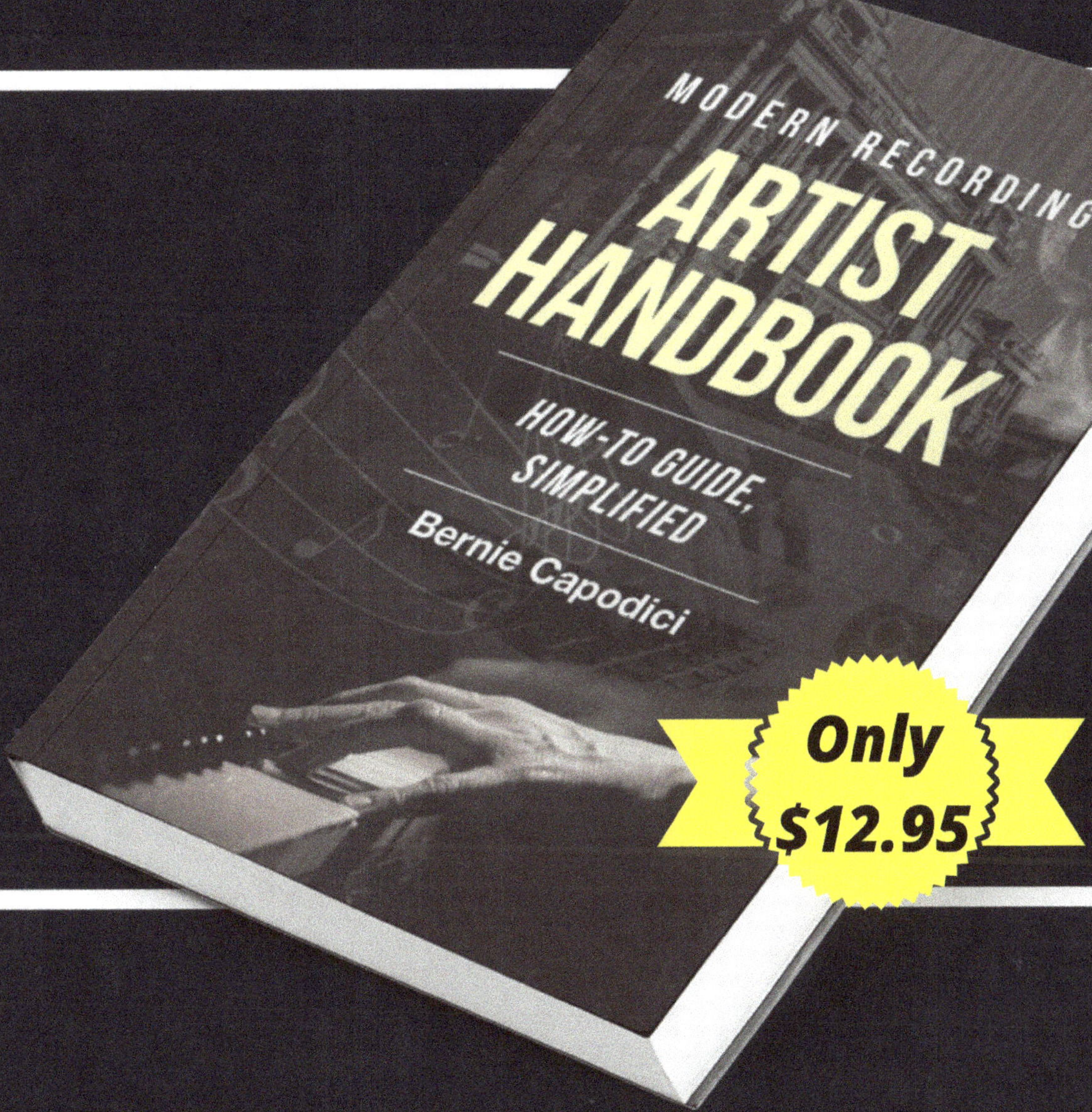

Only $12.95

MUST READ FOR INDEPENDENT ARTISTS

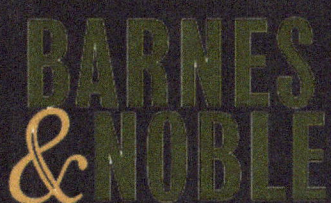

KINDLE $9.99 - HARDCOVER $22.95 - PAPERBACK $12.95

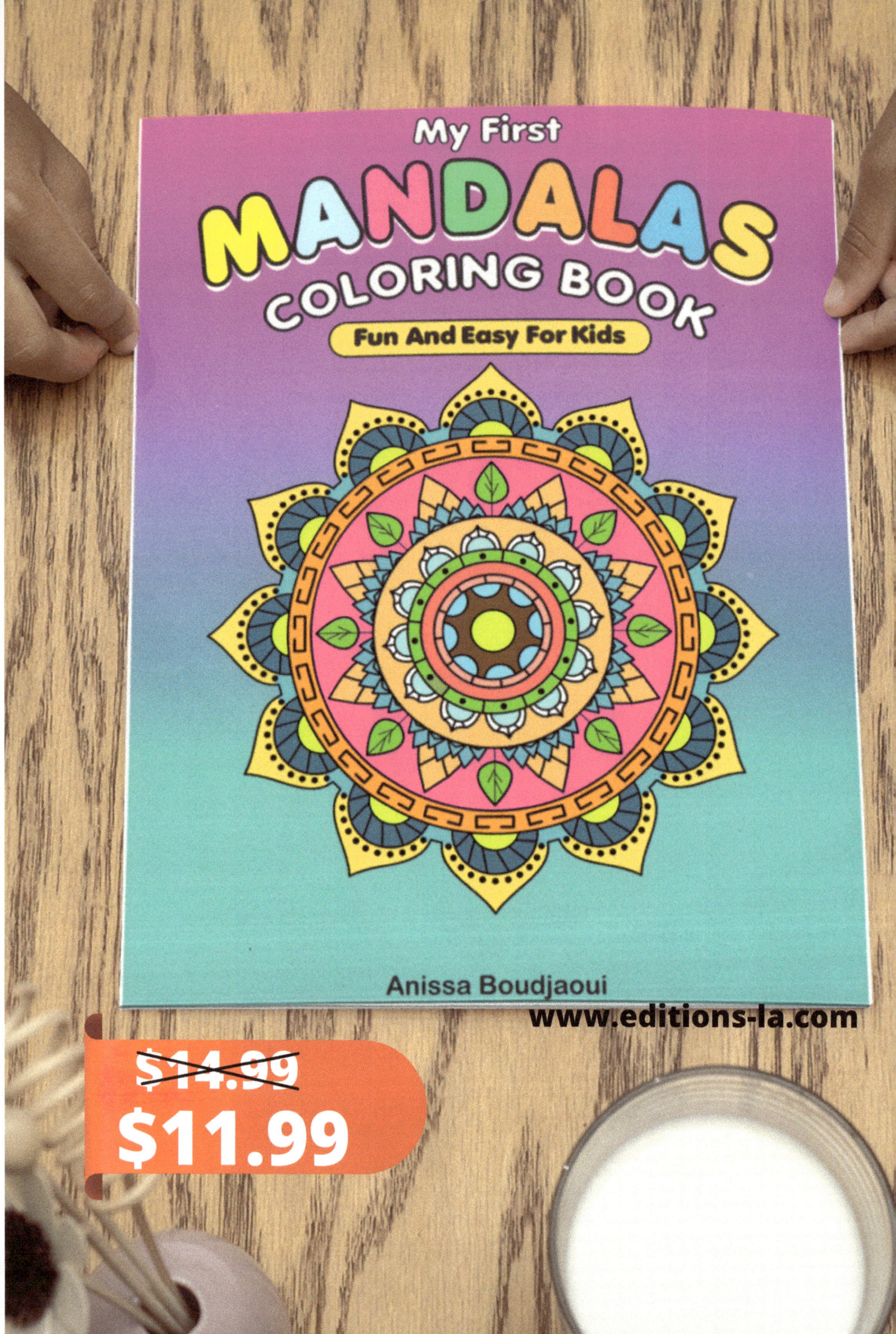

SUMMER 2021
SHADES, SHOES, DRESSES

As we go back in time with fashion, lots of the new summer 2021 trends are inspired by our favorite decades. Today, we will share three pieces that you need to add in your wardrobe to stay stylish.

KNOT SANDALS

A bonus of these cute knot sandals: Hopefully no one ever steps on you when you're in them, but should someone accidentally take a step backwards, the cushion straps will give your feet a little protection.
Mango
mango.com
$79.99

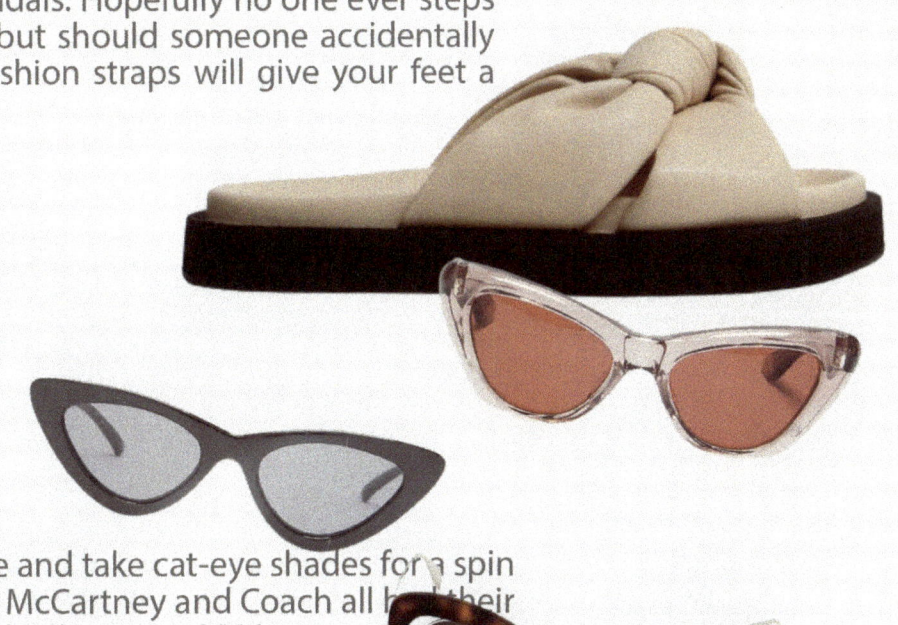

RETRO CAT-EYE SHADES

Embrace your inner '50s muse and take cat-eye shades for a spin this summer. Valentino, Stella McCartney and Coach all had their takes on the retro style for spring/summer 2021, each injecting a contemporary twist to the retro shape.

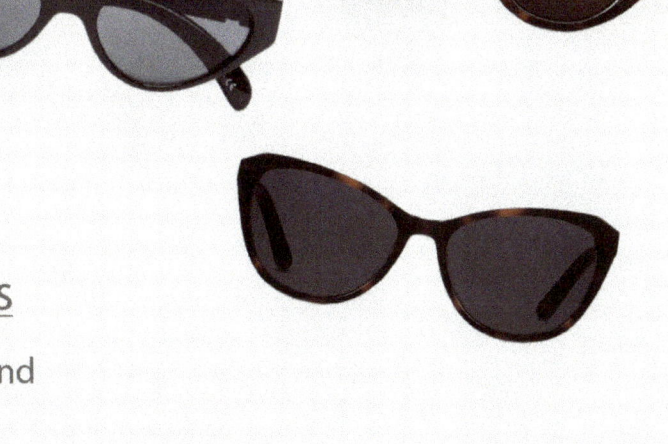

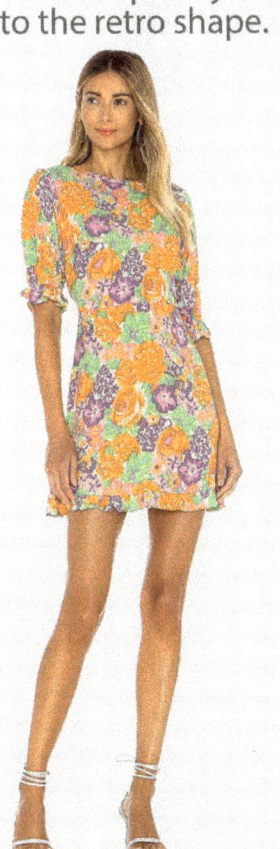

SUMMER DRESS

Faithfull the Brand
revolve.com
$159.00

We love this high-neck minidress with voluminous sleeves and delicate frill detailing. It pairs perfectly with a mini shoulder bag and a pair of strappy sandals.

READ MORE ON
WWW.PUMPITUPMAGAZINE.COM

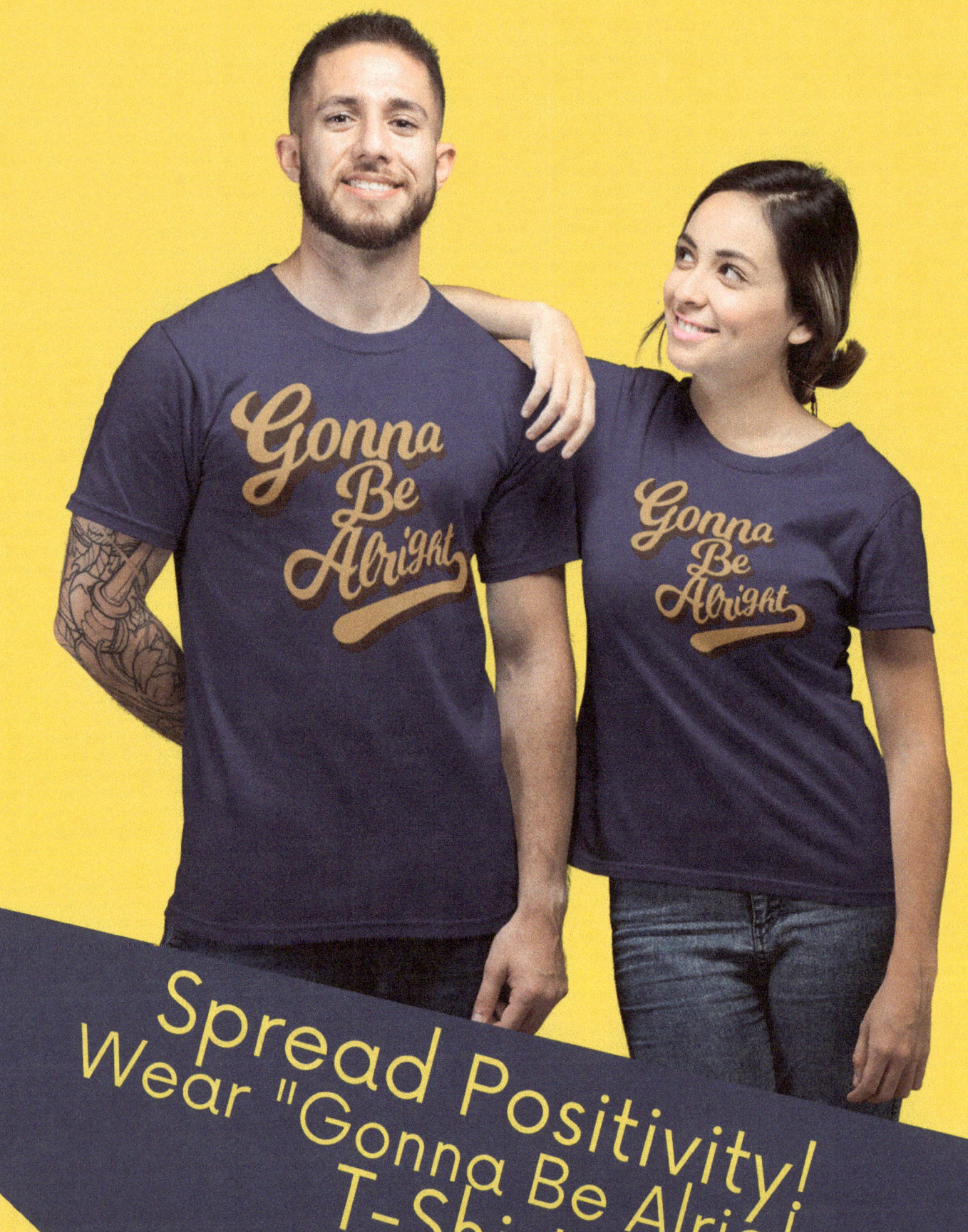

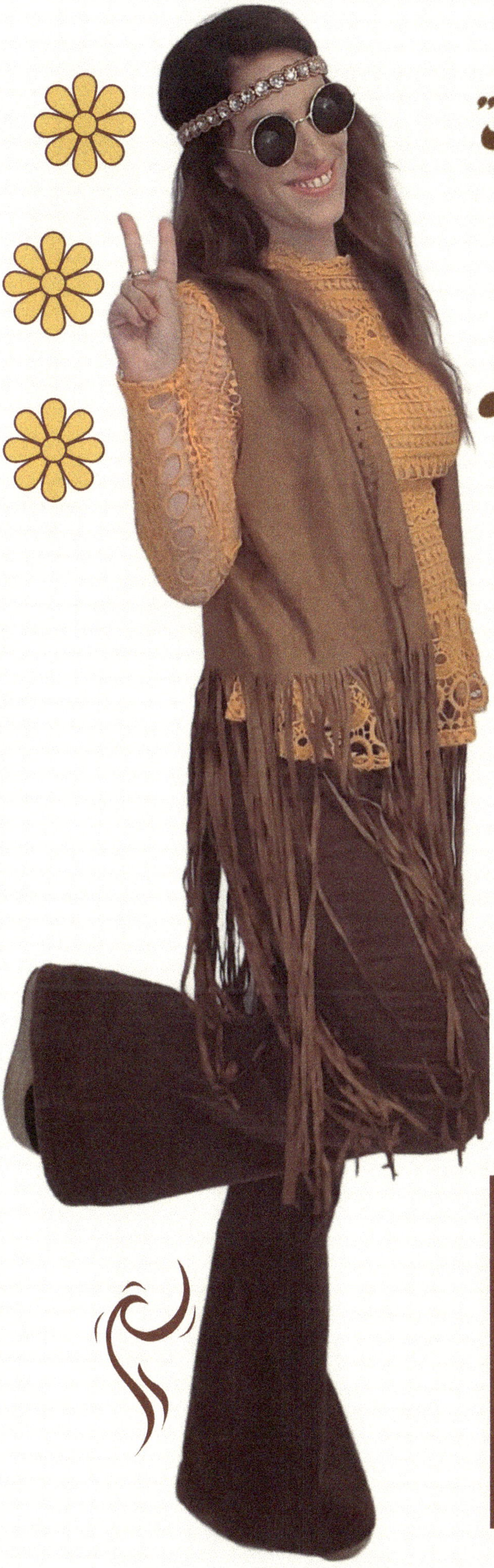

"Dust off your bell bottoms & Let's party like it's 1976!"

Aneessa

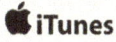 Spotify amazon iTunes
TIDAL

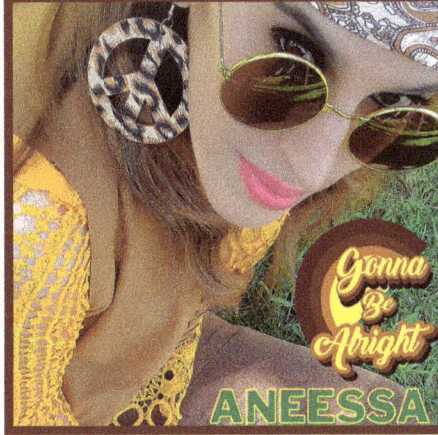

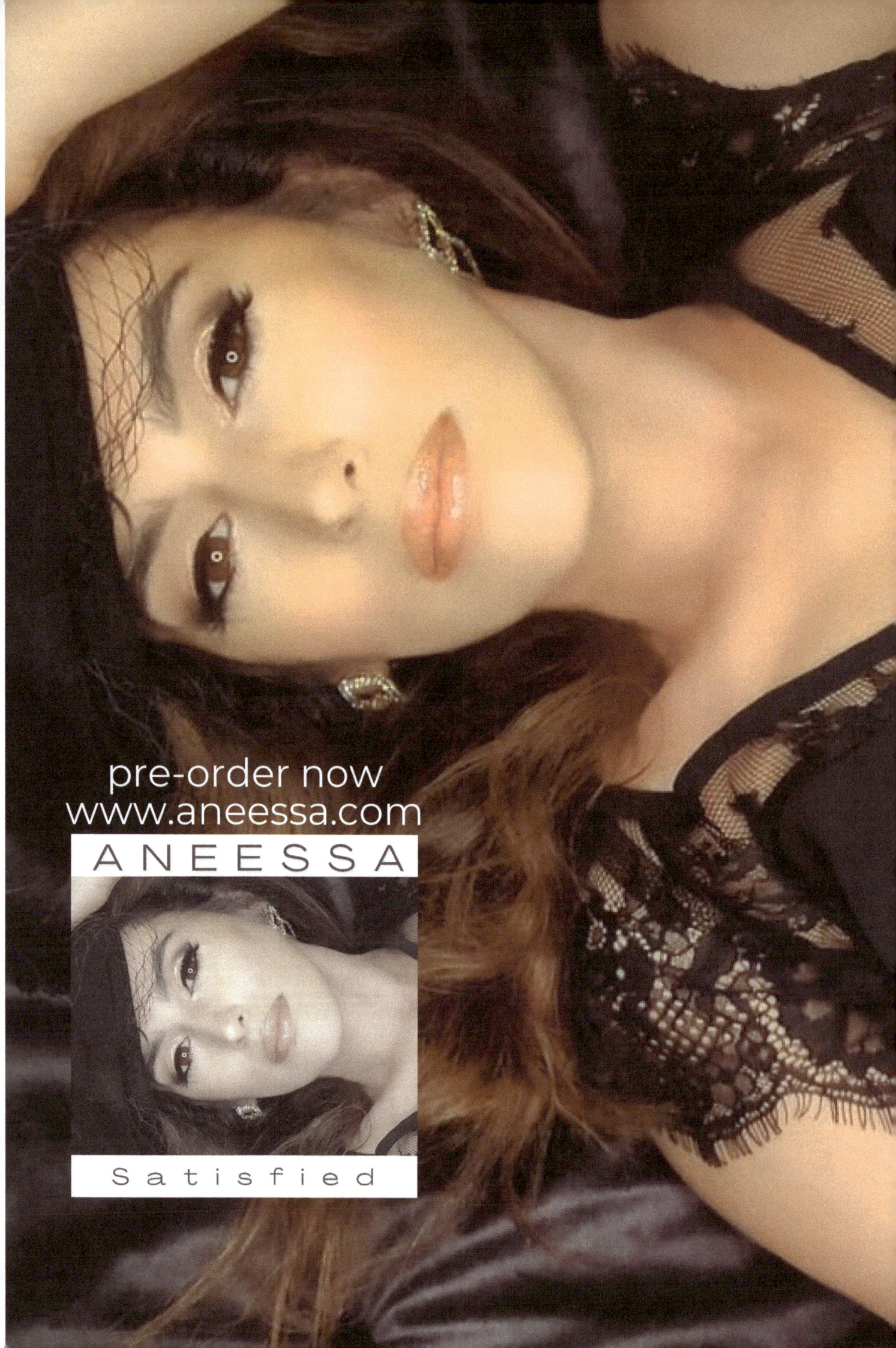

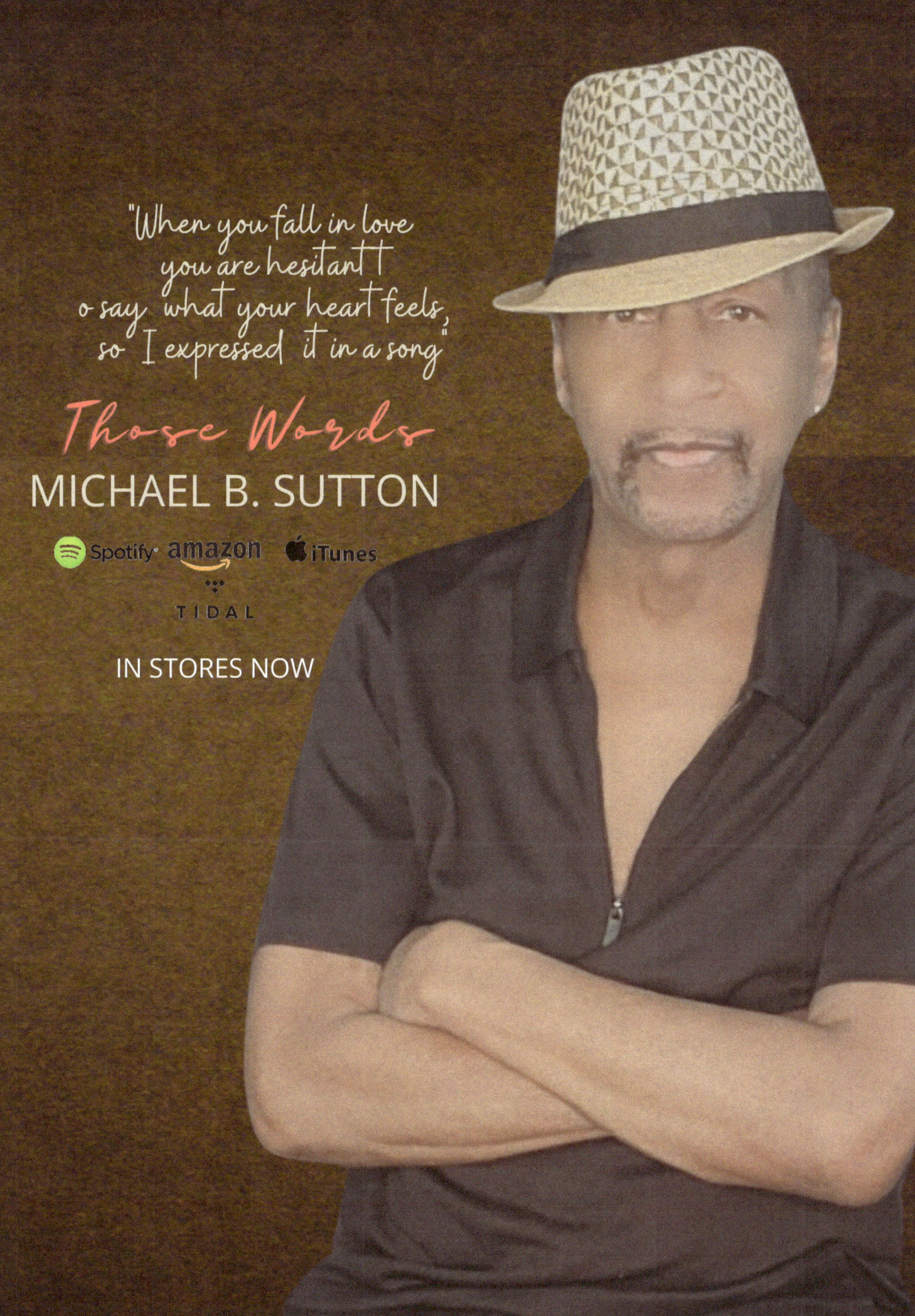

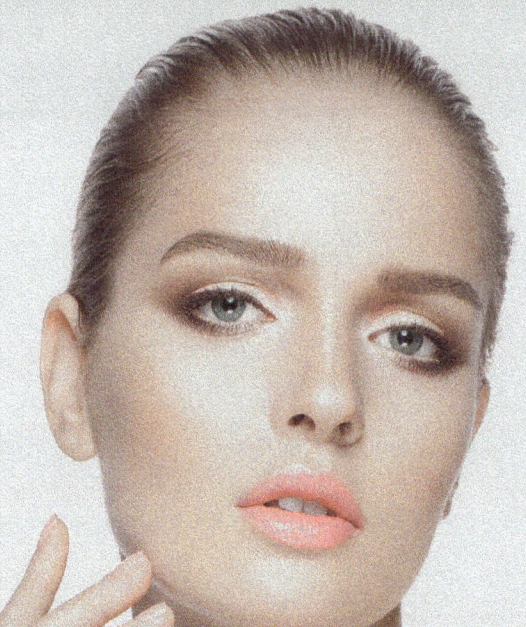

WHAT IS MICRONEEDLING FACIAL?

EVERYTHING YOU NEED TO KNOW

Microneedling. The minimally invasive treatment can be used all over the body—from scalp to ankles—to improve the appearance of scars, boost collagen, or encourage hair growth. Microneedling creates microscopic punctures in the skin.

MICRONEEDLING STIMULATES DORMANT HAIR FOLLICLES.

The stimulation of dormant hair follicles equals new hair growth, confirms Gohara. In a recent study, 100 test subjects were divided into two groups. One set was treated with minoxidil lotion, and the other received minoxidil lotion plus microneedling. After 12 weeks, 82 percent of the microneedling group reported a 50 percent improvement versus 4.5 percent of the minoxidil lotion-only group.

MICRONEEDLING CAN ALSO WORK TO REDUCE CELLULITE.

Alexiades works with a new crop of microneedling devices like the Profound by Candela. She uses the machine for crepe-like fine lines as well as sagging skin and cellulite.

YOUR DERMAROLLER PLAYS WELL WITH OTHER SKINCARE TREATMENTS.

Alexiades recommends pairing microneedling with topical treatments (like her 37 Extreme Actives anti-aging cream or serum) and lasers. "Often, we use this as an opportunity to apply anti-aging preparations that will penetrate better through the needle punctures. When you combine with topicals, you have a shot at some collagen building. When combined with radiofrequency, you can see tissue tightening over months," she says.

YOU NEED TO BE GENTLE ON YOUR SKIN AFTER MICRONEEDLING.

"Let the skin chill after microneedling," Gohara says. "For the rest of the day, don't wash the skin, expose it to high heat, sweat too much (that means no sun, no gym, no hot yoga)."

MICRONEEDLING ALONE ONLY GIVES TEMPORARY RESULTS.

Dr. Alexiades notes that a recent AAD study showed that microneeedling alone can only give temporary results that do not last. "As my over ten years of research has shown, you must combine microneedles with radiofrequency to get long term wrinkle and scar reductions and improvements in skin quality," explains Alexiades.

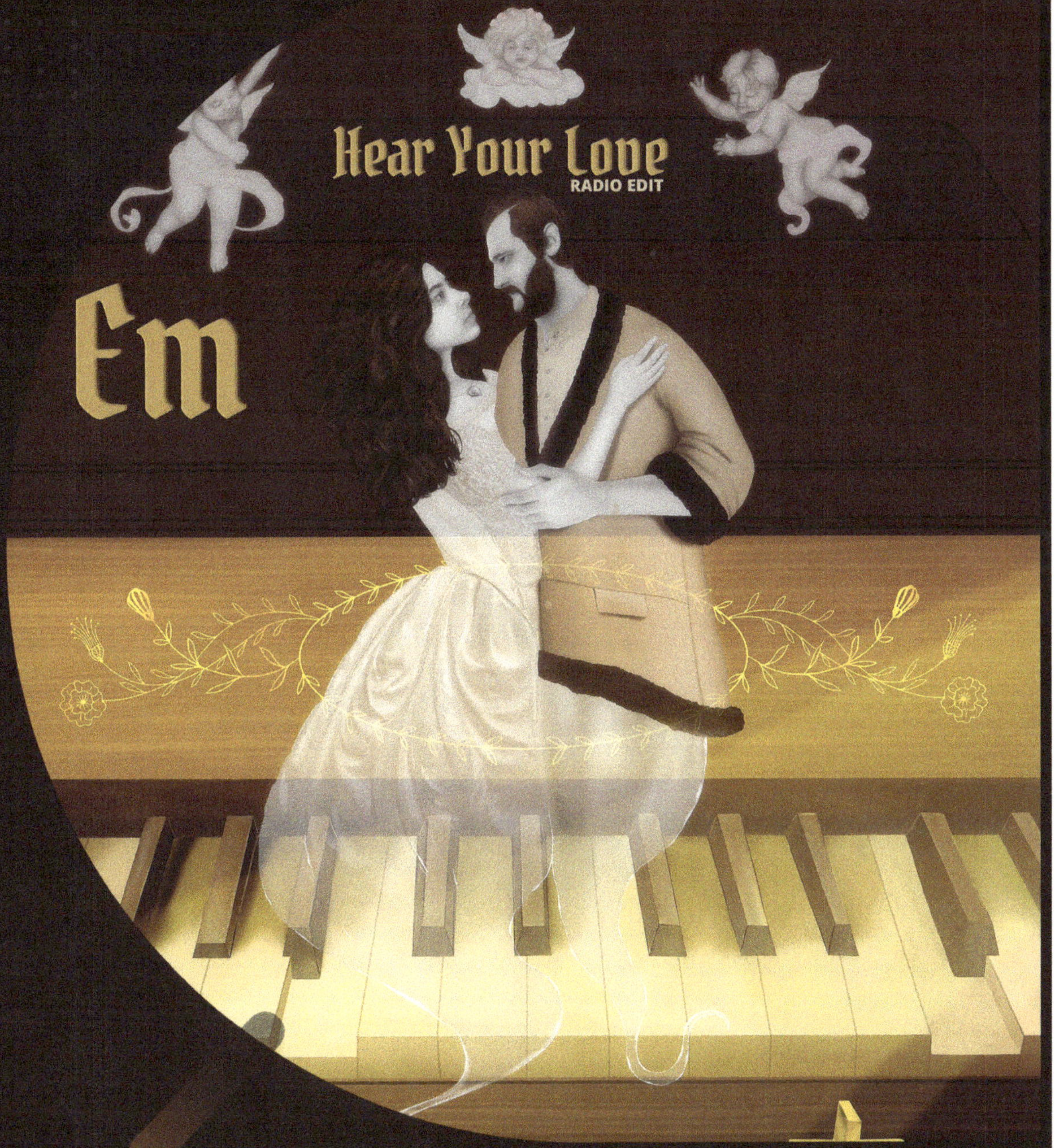

Em
Hear Your Love

Slickly produced, "Hear Your Love" is modern, yet possesses classic cues as well. Anyone with a heart and a memory of love, could blast this track without skipping a beat. The lyrics are relatable enough to let the emotion spill out of the speakers and stand on their own. Moreover, there is a graceful and soulful uniqueness to Em's vocals that make her a timeless talent. Her style is slick, with a domineering depth that often leaves one spellbound, and her songs on replay.

www.Em4Yoursoul.com.com

   @Em4Yoursoul.com

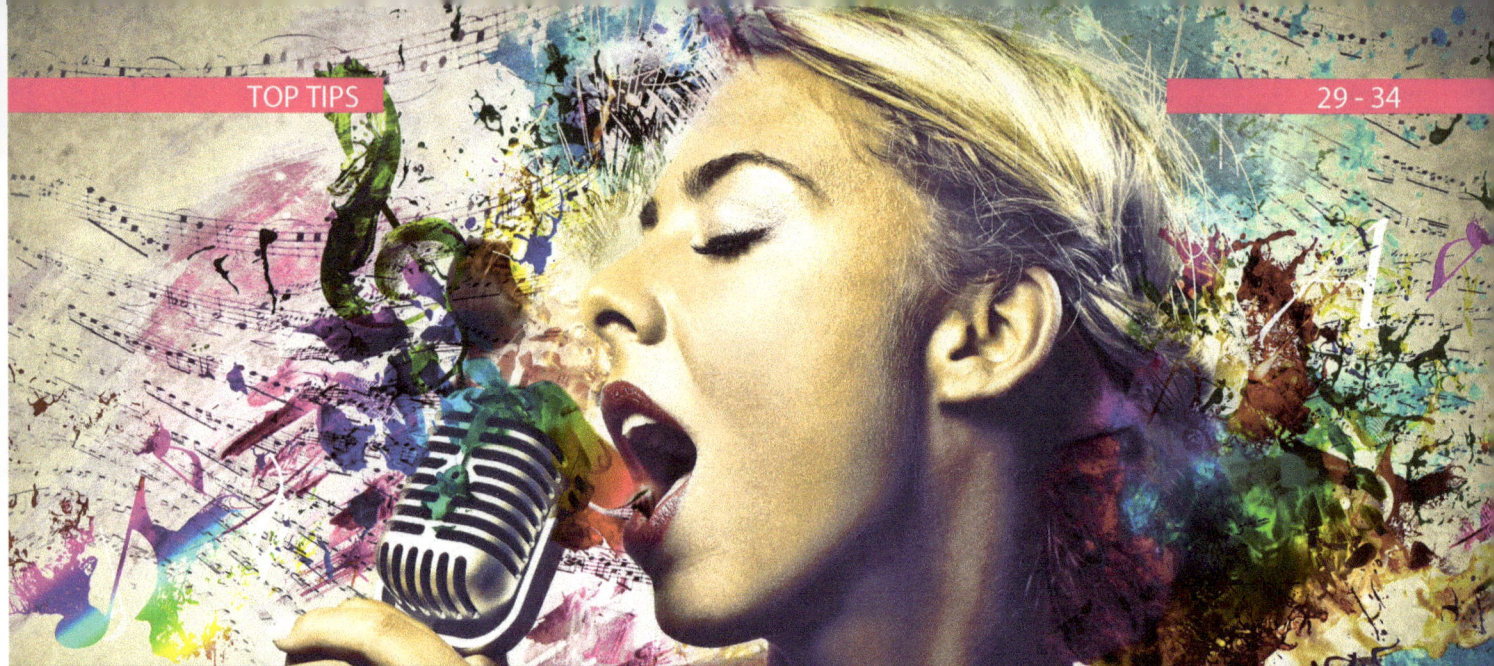

HOW TO BECOME A BETTER SINGER
EVERYTHING YOU NEED TO KNOW

1. WARM UP YOUR BODY BEFORE YOUR VOICE.

Aerobic exercise is a great way to warm up before singing. When your body is energized, your voice responds faster. You'll know you're warm when you start to sweat.

2. RELEASE TENSION.

Tension is a singer's worst enemy. Yoga or deep stretching before you sing will show you where you're holding tension. Don't hold your breath and try to push past your limit. Gently exhale deeper into each stretch. Your mouth and jaw should open and close freely, your facial muscles, lips, tongue, neck, and shoulders should move without tension, and your eyes should be relaxed and alive.

3. HIGH NOTES GO DOWN, NOT UP!

When you approach a high note, think that it goes down, not up! It's like the way a seesaw works. When someone sits on one end, it goes down but your end goes up. The heavier they are, the higher you go. Likewise, give your high notes plenty of oomph "down" if you want them to pop up on the other end.

4. WARM DOWN.

Try humming on low pitches or sliding from your highest, easily reached note, down to your lowest note for a few minutes to warm down after a performance. These exercises re-lubricate tired vocal folds and have a calming effect..

5. SPEAK ON PITCH.

Singing should feel the same as speaking. Rest your fingertips on your Adam's apple (or where it would be for women). This is your larynx which houses your vocal cords. Swallow and it moves up. Yawn and it comes down. When you speak normally it stays in place, even when the spoken pitch varies. The same thing should happen when you sing. It stays still whether you're moving up or down in pitch. Relax your larynx to keep it steady and sing the way you speak.

MUST WATCH

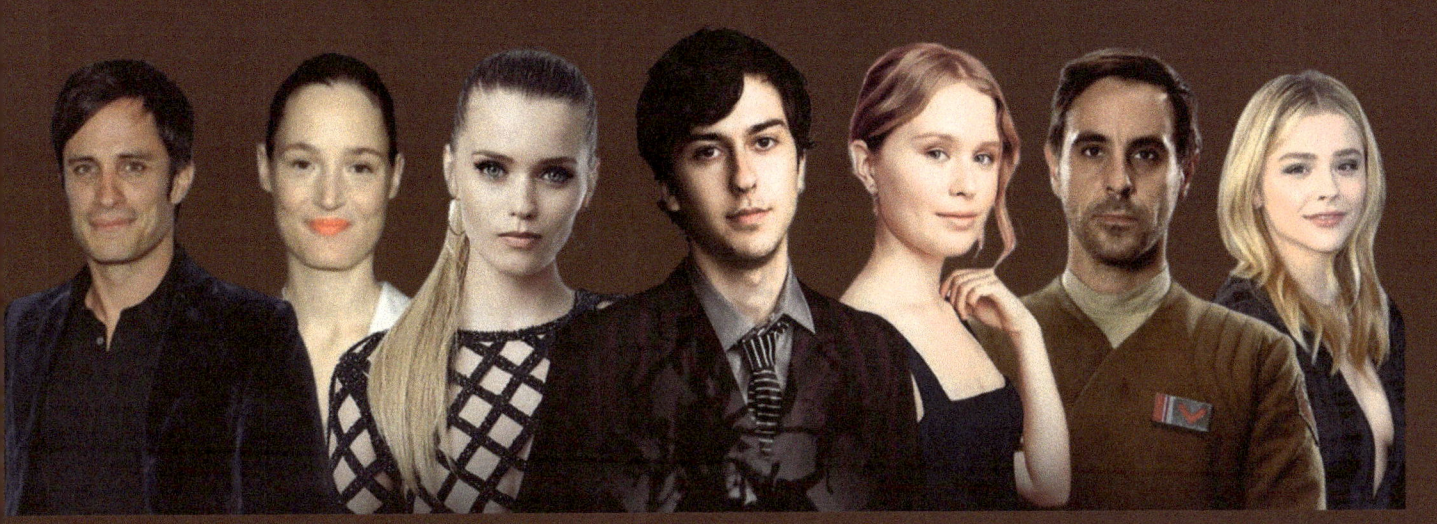

M. NIGHT SHYAMALAN'S NEW MOVIE OLD INSPIRED BY CREEPY GRAPHIC NOVEL ABOUT AGING

M. Night Shyamalan has another creepy story up his sleeve — an entire graphic novel, in fact. Over the weekend, the veteran filmmaker confirmed on Twitter that he's in production on his follow-up to 2019's Glass, writing: "Feels like a miracle that I am standing here shooting the first shot of my new film. It's called Old."

Save for some early artwork, which you can view below, Shyamalan is keeping mum on the details as he's wont to do. However, Collider reports that Old is inspired by Pierre Oscar Lévy and Frederik Peeters' 2010 terrifying graphic novel Sandcastle. The gist of the story involves 13 people who rapidly age on a remote beach.

Here's the full synopsis via Booklist:

By a tidal pool near a small beach on France's Mediterranean coast, a North African–looking man glimpses a young woman stripping to swim. Later, but still early in the morning, three families intent on sunbathing and picnicking encounter the man, then find the girl's corpse in the pool. One paterfamilias, a racist, xenophobic physician, angrily accuses the North African of murder and calls the cops. While awaiting the police, the doctor's mother dies.

The young children of two of the families start growing, the little ones right out of their swimsuits and the preteens into puberty. The adults are changing, too. Attempts to leave the area prove futile, and further calls don't go through. At the rate they're aging, they'll all be dead by tomorrow morning.

Peeters' accomplished European realist comics style and Lévy's utterly natural dialogue suit to a tee this maximally eerie, unsettlingly plein air exercise that Kafkaesquely defies all explanation.

CAST AND CHARACTERS OF OLD

There are many main cast and characters are there in this film they are Rufus Sewell, Abby Lee, Thomasin McKenzie, Embeth Davidtz, Eliza Scanlen, Ken Leung, Alex Wolff, Gael Garcia Bernal, Vicky Krieps, Nikki Amuka Bird, Emun Elliot, Kathleen Chalfant, Matthew Shear, Aaron Pierre, Nolan River, Daniel Ison acted as Greg Mitchel and many other members are also included in this film.

Initially, it was set to release on 26th February 2021 but it was delayed due to this coronavirus pandemic situation. This film has rescheduled and it has set to be released on 23rd July 2021.

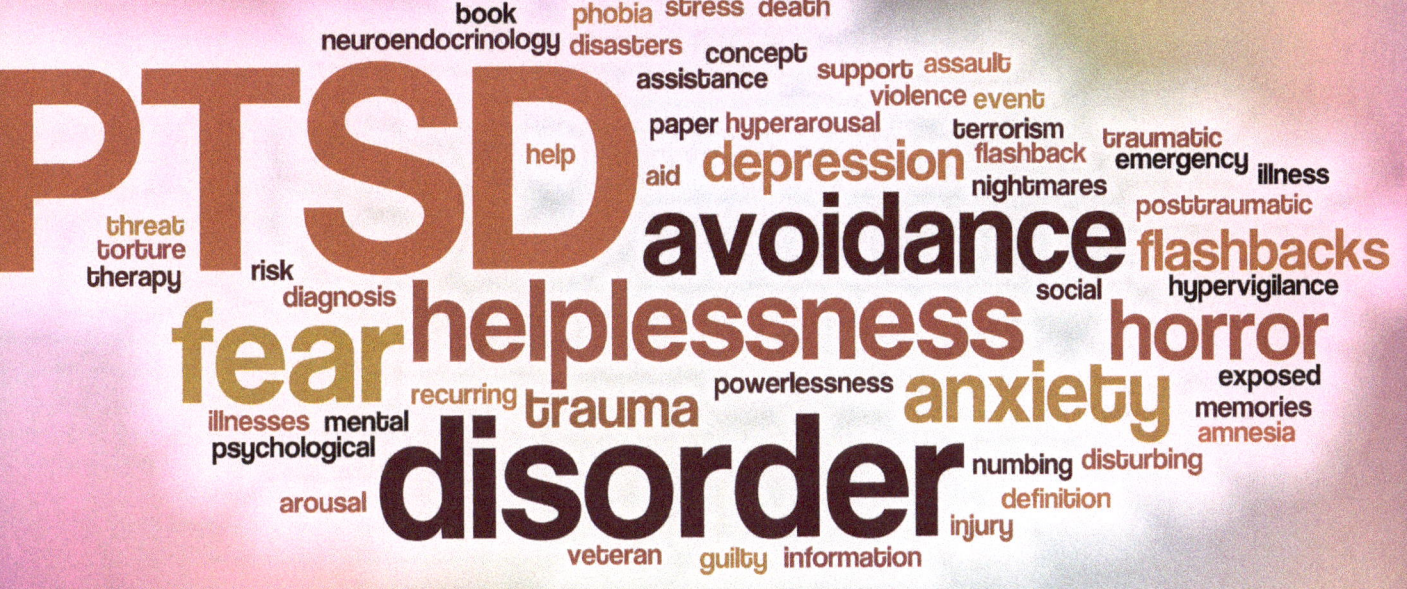

HELP RAISE PTSD AWARENESS
POST TRAUMATIC DISORDER

Post-traumatic stress disorder (PTSD) involves a collection of symptoms that develop in people who have experienced or witnessed a life-threatening trauma such as combat, sexual assault, a serious accident, or a natural disaster.

Common symptoms include feeling on edge, avoiding things that could remind someone of their trauma, flashbacks, and nightmares. This mental health issue has been misunderstood in the past as a sign of weakness or something that cannot be cured, but that is not the case.

WHAT IS PTSD & WHY IS IT IMPORTANT?

People with PTSD often have difficulty getting close to others. This issue can negatively impact their friendships, marriage, or other personal relationships and may leave them feeling unfulfilled because they are not fully engaged in life. PTSD can also lead to other mental health issues such as anxiety and depression. Some people may even abuse drugs or alcohol and eventually require addiction treatment.

Unfortunately, some individuals still hold the misguided belief that PTSD is a form of mental weakness that can be overcome with time and determination. This belief prevents people who are struggling from getting the PTSD treatment they need. As a result, symptoms will likely get worse as a person continues to follow negative patterns rather than resolving the issue.

PTSD Awareness Day looks to change that. The holiday brings to light the silent struggle of millions of Americans and teaches the public that PTSD is a real mental disorder that can be treated. This movement can help encourage people with PTSD to ask for help without shame.

Learning about PTSD can be a starting point for someone who is suffering from it to seek help. It can also be a way for someone who knows nothing about it to be more sympathetic and encouraging to those who struggle.

If you or someone you care about has PTSD, the time is now to take action. Reach out to https://vertavahealth.com/

SPREADING THE WORD ON PTSD

There are many ways to spread the word on PTSD
Even small actions can make a big impact in informing people about PTSD and available treatment options.

WAYS TO ENCOURAGE PTSD AWARENESS MAY INCLUDE:

sharing social media posts or videos about PTSD
leaving posters or pamphlets in public places
organizing a community event to support PTSD treatment
talking to a Veteran about mental health care
sharing resources for people with PTSD
supporting the National Center for PTSD
volunteering with organizations that work with PTSD
educating yourself about PTSD and treatment options

SIGNS SOMEONE NEEDS ADDICTION CARE

Addiction can happen to anyone. What may start as recreational drug use, prescription drug misuse, or binge drinking, can quickly turn into addiction. Often the first step to recovery is realizing that someone needs help.

COMMON SIGNS OF ADDICTION AND SUBSTANCE ABUSE INCLUDE:

Taking drugs/drinking for longer than intended or in larger amounts
Craving or urges to use the substance
Prioritizing drugs or alcohol and neglecting responsibilities or loved ones
Continuing to use the substance even after experiencing negative consequences
Developing a tolerance to the substance
Experiencing withdrawal symptoms when the effects of the substance wears off
Although someone may be exhibiting all these signs of addiction, many people do not get alcohol or drug addiction treatment because they are in denial or afraid to come forward. For some getting substance use disorder treatment requires a drug intervention or court-ordered rehab.

DON'T WAIT. GET HELP NOW
TEL: 844-451-0325

HTTPS://VERTAVAHEALTH.COM/

205 Reidhurst Ave | Nashville, TN 37203
1 (833) VERTAVA

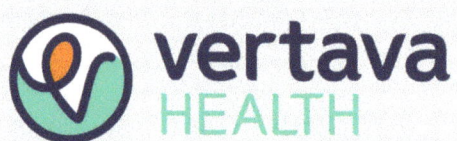

info@vertavahealth.com

www.ingramcontent.com/pod-product-compliance
Lightning Source LLC
Chambersburg PA
CBHW051810010526
44118CB00024BA/2819